FENNEL

MARIAN KIM

CONTENTS

MARIAN KIM

1

PROPERTIES

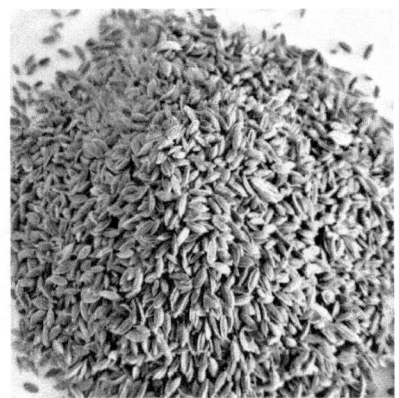

Scientific name: Foeniculum vulgare

Other names: Fennel seed, sweet fennel, fenkel

Nutrients: Fennel contains vitamins B3 (niacin), B5 (pantothenic acid), B9 (folate), C. It also contains mineral like calcium, copper, iron, magnesium, manganese, molybdenum, phosphorus, potassium. Fennel also contains phytoestrogens and fiber.

Properties

Appetite suppressant

Antioxidant properties which protect the cells from the free radical damage that causes premature aging and degenerative diseases.

Anti-cancer properties

Anti-spasmodic properties

Carminative (anti-flatulent) properties

Diuretic (increases urine production) properties

Emmenagogue (stimulate menstrual flow) properties

Estrogen-like properties in the body

Expectorant properties

Galactagogue (stimulate breast milk production) properties

* * * * *

2

USES

Insomnia treatment

Fennel helps relieve insomnia or sleeplessness.

Flatulence treatment and prevention

Fennel tea is used to treat flatulence (intestinal gas) and bloating. It also helps prevent excessive wind.

Colic treatment

Fennel is used to treat colic in infants.

Heartburn treatment

Fennel is used to treat heartburn.

Cholera treatment

Fennel is used to treat cholera. Fennel tea is also used for food poisoning.

Irritable bowels

Fennel tea is used for irritable bowels since it relaxes the smooth muscles lining the digestive tract.

Halitosis treatment

Fennel tea can be used as gargle to reduce halitosis (bad breath) since it has a fresh, aromatic scent and it aids with the digestive process.

Coughs treatment

Fennel is used to treat coughs and other upper respiratory tract infections since it has expectorant properties. See recipe for fennel syrup below.

Asthma treatment

Fennel is used for asthma. It is also used for bronchitis and respiratory congestion since it has expectorant properties.

Nasal congestion treatment

1 tablespoon of fennel seeds can be added to 1 pint (500 ml) of boiling water and the vapor inhaled to ease nasal congestion.

Sore throat relief

Fennel tea can be gargled 3 times a day to relieve sore throats.

Breath freshener

Fennel freshens the breath.

Backache treatment

Fennel is used to treat backaches.

Breast enlargement

Fennel is used for breast enlargement.

Breast milk induction

Fennel is used to increase the production of breast milk. However, it has been reported that some breast-feeding infants experienced damage to their nervous system after their mothers drunk herbal teas with fennel.

Menstruation induction

Fennel is used to treat amenorrhea (lack of periods) since it promotes menstruation. Fennel tea can also be used to relieve the symptoms of PMS.

Menopausal symptom relief

Fennel tea can be used to manage the symptoms of menopause since it has estrogen-like effects in the body.

Birthing

Fennel is used to ease the birthing process.

Poor libido

Fennel is used to boost libido and increase the sex drive in women.

Bedwetting

Fennel is used for bedwetting.

Weight loss

Fennel tea is used for weight loss since it suppresses the appetite especially if it is drunk 15 minutes before a meal.

Water retention and kidney disorders

Fennel is used for water retention and other kidney disorders since it increases urine flow.

Liver and spleen disorders

Fennel is used for liver and spleen disorders.

Angina treatment

Fennel is used for angina.

Anxiety and depression

Fennel is used for anxiety and depression.

Snake bite relief

Fennel poultice is used for snake bites.

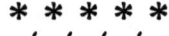

3

SAFETY PRECAUTIONS

1. Persons with hormone-sensitive conditions like cancers of the breast, uterus and ovaries as well as condition like uterine fibroids and endometriosis should not use fennel since it has estrogen-like properties in the body.

2. People who are allergic to celery, carrots and mugwort can develop allergic reactions to fennel.

3. Fennel can make the skin more sensitive to sunlight and thus increase the chances of a person developing sunburn and skin cancer. Light skinned persons should therefore apply sunscreen when using fennel.

4. Due to its phytoestrogen properties fennel is not recommended for pregnant women.

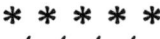

4

DRUG INTERACTIONS

1. Women taking oral contraceptives (birth control pills) with estrogens should not use/avoid fennel since it has estrogen-like properties and it might decrease the effectiveness of the pills. They can also use additional birth control like condoms.

2. Women taking hormone replacement therapy (HRT) with estrogens like conjugated equine estrogens (Premarin) should not use/avoid fennel since it has estrogen-like properties and it might decrease the effectiveness of the HRT.

3. Persons taking tamoxifen (Nolvadex) should not use fennel since it might decrease its effectiveness.

4. Persons taking ciprofloxacin (Cipro) should not use/avoid fennel since it might decrease its effectiveness.

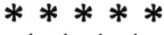

6

HERBAL RECIPES

Basic Fennel Tea

Equipment

Kettle

Tea cup

***

Ingredients

1 teaspoon of finely crushed fennel

1 cup of boiling water

Honey to taste (optional)

***

Instructions

1. Put the fennel in a tea cup, add the boiling water and let it steep while covered for 10 -15 minutes.

2. Add honey (if using) to suit your taste before drinking.

***

Tips

1. Bruise the fennel in a mortar with a pestle before adding the boiling water to help them release their oils.

2. This tea can be drunk to increase breast milk production by lactating mothers. It can also be used as a gargle for sore throats and to freshen the breath.

*****

Fennel Flatulence Treatment Tea

Equipment

Tea pot

***

Ingredients

1 teaspoon fennel, 1 teaspoon anise, 1 teaspoon caraway, 1 teaspoon coriander seeds

4 cups of boiling water

***

Instructions

1. Put the fennel, anise, caraway and coriander seeds in the teapot, add the boiling water and let it steep while covered for 10 -15 minutes before drinking.

*****

Fennel Colic Water

Equipment
Tea pot

***

Ingredients
1 teaspoon fennel

½ teaspoon sugar

1 cup of boiling water

***

Instructions
1. Boil the fennel in the water for 5 minutes.

2. Add the sugar, stir and remove the mixture from the heat source.

3. Strain the fennel and give a teaspoon of the fennel colic water to the baby three times a day.

*****

Fennel Syrup

Equipment
Saucepan

Jar with airtight lid

***

Ingredients
1 quart (1000 ml) filtered water

1 cup fennel

1 cup honey

***

Instructions
1. Place the water and fennel in a saucepan and bring to a boil.

2. Reduce the heat and let it simmer while it is partially covered until the volume is reduced to half the original volume.

3. Strain the mixture through a sieve or cheesecloth to remove the fennel.

4. Measure 1 pint (500 mls) of the liquid and add the honey.

5. Cook for a few minutes as you stir it so that it thickens.

6. Store the syrup in an airtight container in the fridge for up to 2 months.

*****

Fennel Poultice

Equipment

Cheesecloth or old cotton sheet strips

***

Ingredients

1 tablespoon powdered fennel

Boiling water

***

Instructions

1. Add enough boiling water to the fennel to wet it and make a thick paste.

2. Spoon the fennel paste onto the cheesecloth (or bed sheet strips) to make the poultice.

3. To use, apply the poultice to the affected area and cover with another piece of hot, wet cloth. Replace the hot, wet cloth when it cools with another hot one to keep the poultice hot.

*****

Fennel Tincture

Equipment

Glass jar with tight fitting lid

Dark tincture bottles

Cheesecloth

Labels

***

Ingredients

7 oz (200 gm) of fennel

30 oz (1 liter) of 80-100 proof vodka

***

Instructions

1. Fill 1/3 of the glass jar with the chopped fennel.

2. Add the vodka to completely fill the jar to the top.

3. Seal the jar, label it and store it in a dark place for 6 weeks ensuring that you shake them weekly.

4. After 6 weeks strain out the fennel with a cheesecloth and pour the tincture into dark tincture bottles.

5. Label the tincture bottles with the date and name of fennel used and store your herbal tinctures away from light and heat.

*****

Fennel Infused Oil

Equipment

Double boiler

Large glass bowl

Sieve and cheesecloth

Sterilized dark jars

***

Ingredients

16 fl oz. (500 ml) vegetable oil like olive or sweet almond oil

8 oz. (250 grams) slightly crushed fennel

***

Instructions

1. Place the fennel and oil in the glass bowl ensuring that the oil covers the fennel. Simmer them in a double boiler for 1 hour at a temperature of around 120 degrees Fahrenheit (49 degrees Celsius). Do not let the mixture boil. You can repeat this step several times after letting the oils cool to create more concentrated herb infused oils.

2. Strain the mixture through the sieve and cheesecloth into a clean, dark jar ensuring you squeeze out as much oil as you can from the cheesecloth.

3. Label your jars with the manufacturing date, expiry date, fennel and oils used.

4. Store your fennel infused oils in a cool dark place or in the refrigerator and use them within 3 months.

*****

Fennel Butter

Equipment

Large glass bowl

Electric mixer or stick blender or wire whisk

Molds such as ice cube trays (optional)

***

Ingredients

½ cup butter

2 tablespoons of finely crushed fennel

***

Instructions

1. Place the butter in a warm place so that it can soften.

2. Put butter and fennel in a large glass bowl and blend well until thoroughly mixed.

3. Refrigerate until it hardens. You can refrigerate it in molds or ice cube trays to give it a special shape.

###

ABOUT THE AUTHOR

Marian Kim is an experienced alternative medicine practitioner.

*****

OTHER BOOKS BY THE AUTHOR

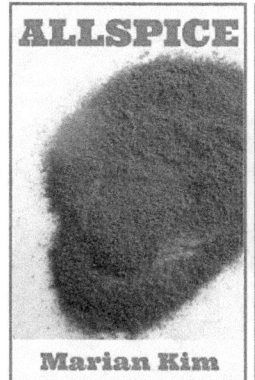

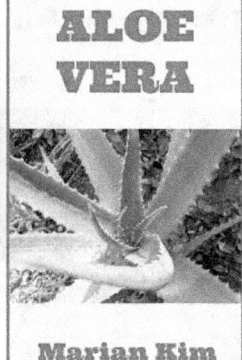

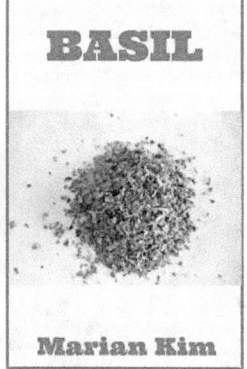

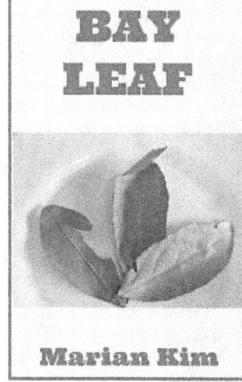

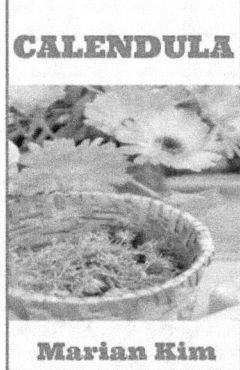

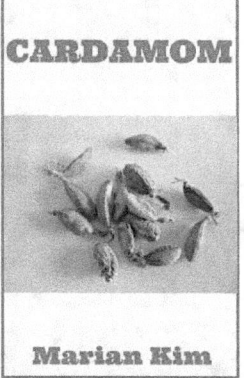

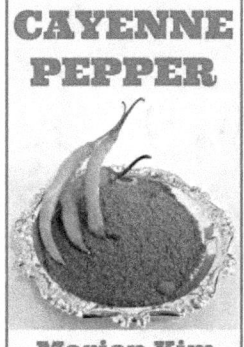

CAYENNE PEPPER

Marian Kim

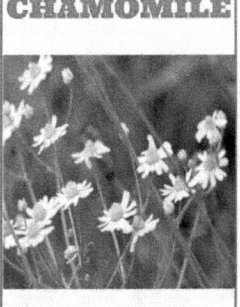

CHAMOMILE

Marian Kim

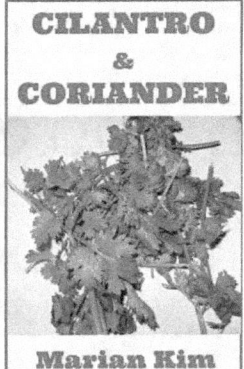

CILANTRO & CORIANDER

Marian Kim

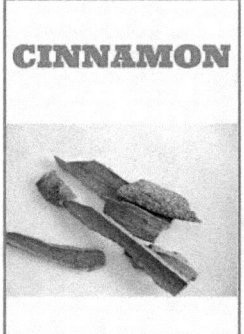

CINNAMON

Marian Kim

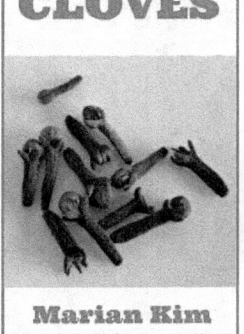

CLOVES

Marian Kim

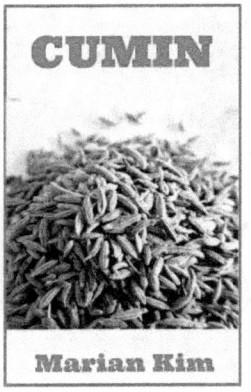

CUMIN

Marian Kim

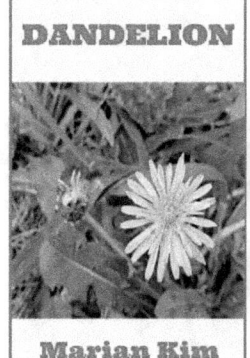

DANDELION

Marian Kim

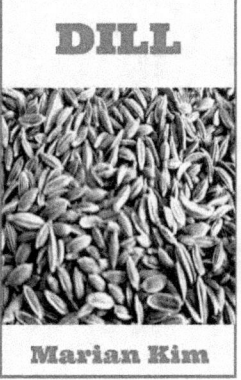

DILL

Marian Kim

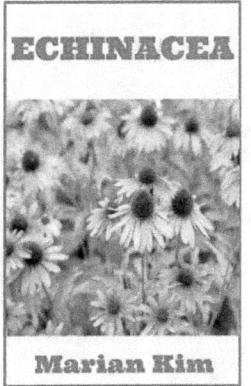

ECHINACEA

Marian Kim

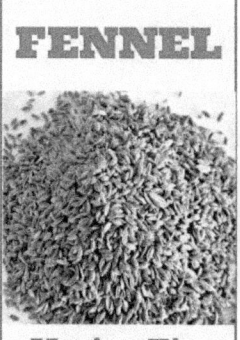

FENNEL

Marian Kim

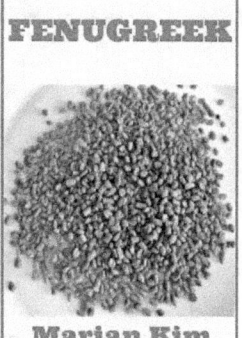

FENUGREEK

Marian Kim

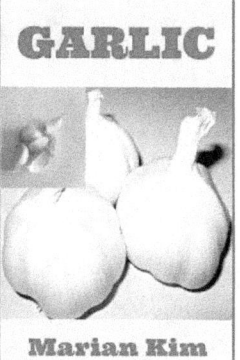

GARLIC

Marian Kim

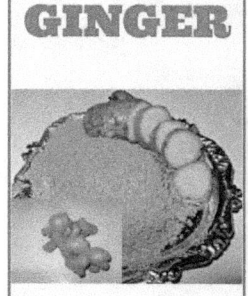

GINGER

Marian Kim

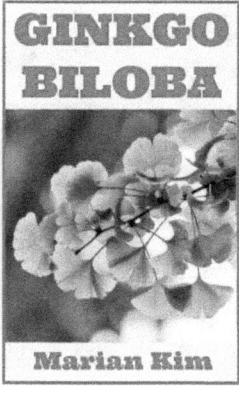

GINKGO BILOBA

Marian Kim

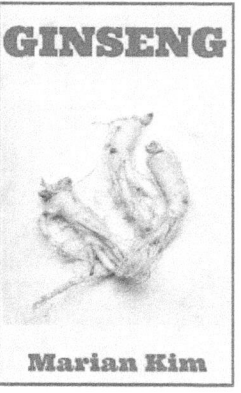

GINSENG

Marian Kim

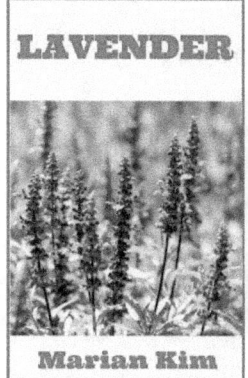

LAVENDER

Marian Kim

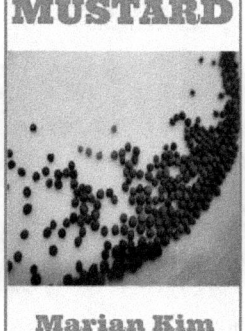

MUSTARD

Marian Kim

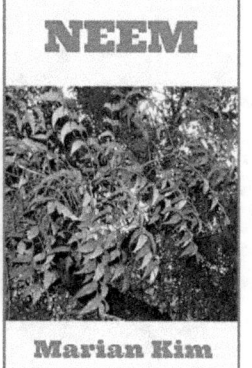

NEEM

Marian Kim

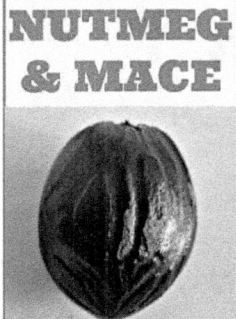

NUTMEG & MACE

Marian Kim

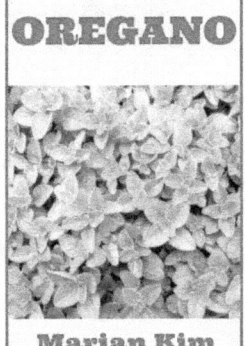

OREGANO

Marian Kim

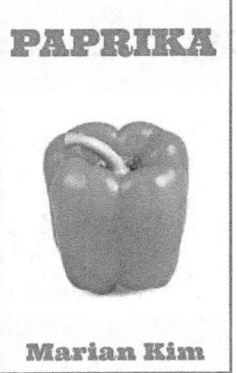

PAPRIKA

Marian Kim

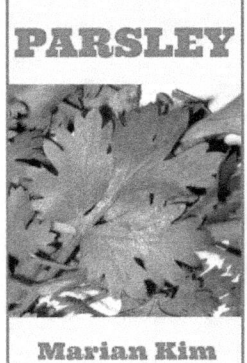

PARSLEY

Marian Kim

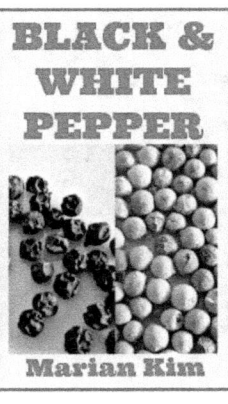

BLACK & WHITE PEPPER

Marian Kim

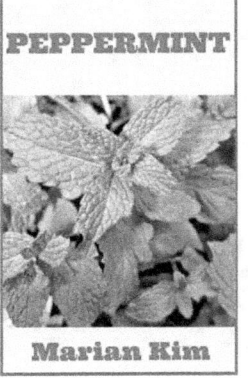

PEPPERMINT

Marian Kim

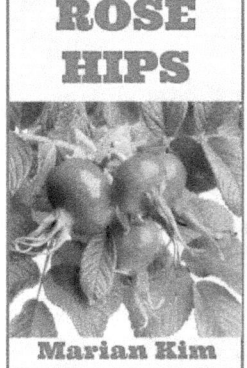

ROSE HIPS

Marian Kim

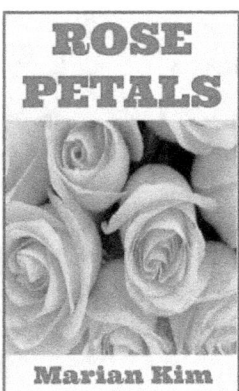

ROSE PETALS

Marian Kim

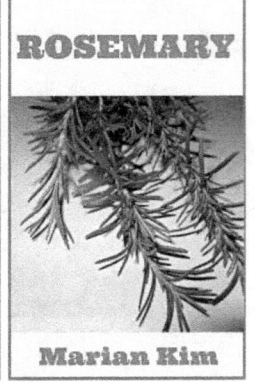

ROSEMARY

Marian Kim

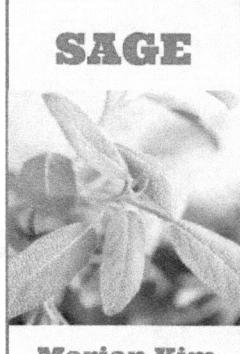

SAGE

Marian Kim

ST. JOHN'S WORT

Marian Kim

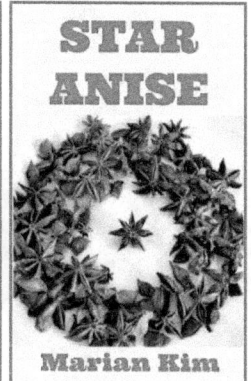

STAR ANISE

Marian Kim

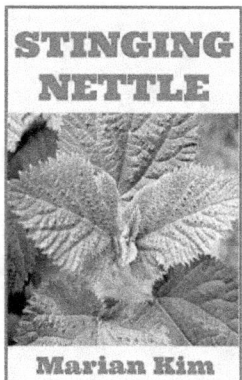

STINGING NETTLE

Marian Kim

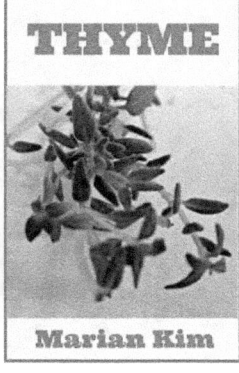

THYME

Marian Kim

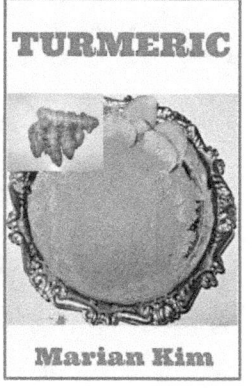

TURMERIC

Marian Kim

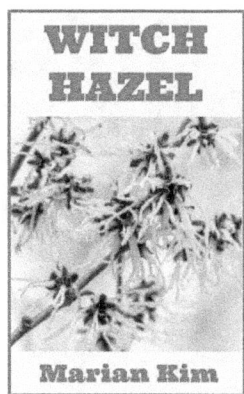

WITCH HAZEL

Marian Kim

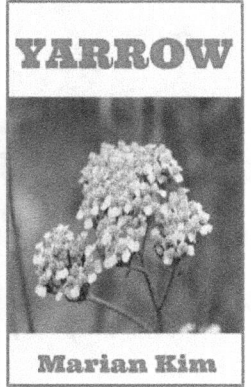

YARROW

Marian Kim

*****